UNDERSTANDING

LASER SKIN RESURFACING TECHNIQUES

FOR BEGINNERS

Unlocking The Secrets To Flawless Skin: Expert Insights On Procedures, Benefits, Aftercare, And Choosing The Right Treatment

DR. ALICIA SONYA

CONTENTS

DISCLAIMER

The information provided in this book is for educational and informational purposes only and is not intended as medical advice, diagnosis, or treatment. Always consult with a qualified healthcare professional before beginning any therapy, practice, or lifestyle change.

The author and publisher of this book make no representations or warranties regarding the accuracy, applicability, or completeness of the content presented. While every effort has been made to ensure the information provided is accurate and up-to-date, the field of health and wellness is constantly evolving, and the reader is advised to use discretion and seek professional guidance as needed.

This book contains references to individuals, products, websites, organizations, or other entities solely for informational purposes. The author and publisher do not endorse, sponsor, or affiliate with any of these references, nor do they receive any benefit from their inclusion. The mention of any names, trademarks, or products does not imply any association or endorsement.

The use of this book is solely at the reader's discretion. Neither the author nor the publisher shall be held liable for any damages, loss, or injury resulting from the use or misuse of the information contained herein.

ABOUT THIS BOOK

Understanding Laser Skin Resurfacing Techniques For Beginners " is designed to be the essential resource for anyone seeking to understand and master the complexities of laser skin resurfacing. This comprehensive guide covers every aspect of laser skin treatment, from the science behind different laser types to the detailed steps of aftercare, making it a valuable tool for practitioners and patients alike. This book begins by laying a foundation with an introductory overview of laser skin resurfacing, covering its purpose, historical evolution, and the types of skin issues that benefit from this advanced technology.

It also identifies who stands to benefit most from these treatments, providing readers with the insights needed to evaluate whether laser resurfacing aligns with their skincare goals.

This guide then delves into the various laser resurfacing techniques, explaining the unique properties and benefits of CO_2 lasers, erbium lasers, and fractional lasers. Each laser type is thoroughly explained in terms of its applications and advantages, enabling readers to make informed decisions about which technique may best suit their skin type and individual concerns. Non-ablative and ablative lasers are discussed in depth, with guidance on how to choose the appropriate option for distinct skincare needs.

Preparing for laser resurfacing is just as critical as the treatment itself, and this book emphasizes the importance of preparation through thorough consultations, skin assessments, and pre-treatment skincare routines. Readers are guided through essential steps such as avoiding certain products, adjusting lifestyle factors, and understanding potential risks. The preparation stage is explained with clarity, ensuring that individuals can approach the treatment confidently and knowledgeably.

Each laser session unfolds in a series of precise steps, and this guide breaks down the entire procedure, from pain management to post-treatment expectations.

By explaining what happens during a session, this book demystifies the experience, offering tips on managing pain and remaining comfortable. Readers can explore the differences in treatment durations for each laser type, gaining a realistic perspective on what to anticipate.

Effective aftercare is vital for maximizing the results of laser resurfacing, and this book outlines best practices for immediate post-treatment care, including recommended skincare routines and product choices. Managing post-procedure side effects like swelling and redness is covered in detail, along with essential advice for avoiding sun exposure.

This book also provides a clear recovery timeline, giving readers a practical framework for tracking their skin's healing journey.

For those curious about how to maintain their results, this guide offers insights into prolonging the effects of laser resurfacing through proper skin care and maintenance treatments. Practical tips for enhancing the longevity of results are shared, helping readers protect their investment in their skin. Recognizing that individual factors can impact how long results last, this book provides tools for readers to tailor maintenance to their needs.

Understanding the potential risks and common concerns of laser skin resurfacing is essential, and this book addresses them directly, covering topics like hyperpigmentation, scarring, and infection prevention. Readers will gain a clear understanding of post-treatment symptoms, from redness and swelling to sensitivity, with actionable steps for managing these effects. Common myths surrounding laser skin resurfacing are dispelled, providing a balanced perspective on what to realistically expect.

Choosing the right clinic and practitioner is critical, and this guide equips readers with tools to find reputable professionals who meet high standards of care.

Tips on verifying credentials, assessing clinic reputation, and recognizing red flags are provided, ensuring readers can make safe and informed decisions when selecting their provider.

Laser skin resurfacing can vary significantly based on skin type, and this guide thoroughly explores how factors like skin tone and sensitivity can affect treatment outcomes. It addresses considerations based on the Fitzpatrick scale and guides tailoring treatments to accommodate different skin textures and conditions, such as acne scars and rosacea.

This book concludes with answers to frequently asked questions, providing clarity on topics such as treatment pain, the ideal age for laser treatments, the potential for combining procedures, and post-treatment guidelines for wearing makeup.

This section serves as a valuable reference, covering the most common questions and concerns to ensure readers feel fully informed and empowered to embark on their laser skin resurfacing journey with confidence.

CHAPTER ONE

Introduction To Laser Skin Resurfacing

Laser skin resurfacing is a popular aesthetic treatment that uses focused beams of light to improve skin texture, tone, and overall appearance. This procedure removes or reshapes the outer layers of skin to reveal smoother, more youthful-looking skin underneath.

It's effective in reducing wrinkles, fine lines, age spots, scars, and other skin irregularities. Laser skin resurfacing can be performed in different intensities and depths, depending on the individual's skin needs, from superficial laser peels to deeper treatments that target more persistent skin issues.

The technology for laser skin treatments began developing in the 1960s with CO_2 lasers. These early lasers were primarily used for medical purposes, but over time, they evolved into aesthetic applications, thanks to advancements that allowed for controlled, precise skin resurfacing. By the 1990s, dermatologists started using lasers specifically to treat wrinkles and scars, and the technology has continued to improve with the introduction of fractional and non-ablative lasers, which offer targeted treatment with minimal downtime.

Laser skin resurfacing addresses a range of skin concerns, including sun damage, fine lines, hyperpigmentation, acne scars, and large pores.

It's beneficial for people with uneven skin tone or texture, and it's often a preferred choice for individuals seeking non-surgical anti-aging treatments.

However, laser resurfacing may be best suited for those with fair to medium skin tones, as certain lasers can cause pigmentation changes in darker skin. Consulting with a dermatologist helps determine if laser resurfacing is suitable for your skin type and goals.

Overview Of Laser Skin Resurfacing And Its Purpose

Laser skin resurfacing aims to improve skin appearance by using precise laser technology to remove damaged or aged skin layers, promoting new skin growth and collagen production.

This treatment can be adjusted for different depths, from light peels that focus on minor imperfections to deep resurfacing for more significant skin issues. The procedure is known for delivering smoother, firmer skin with reduced scars, wrinkles, and pigmentation marks.

The process of laser resurfacing works by directing concentrated beams of light at specific areas of the skin, which heats the layers beneath, stimulating collagen formation. This promotes skin tightening and helps reduce sagging and wrinkles.

Ablative lasers, like CO_2 and Erbium, remove outer layers of skin, while non-ablative lasers penetrate without removing layers, focusing on collagen formation and skin elasticity improvements over time. Choosing the right type of laser depends on skin type, concerns, and desired recovery time.

This treatment is valuable for individuals seeking non-surgical options to address signs of aging, acne scars, or uneven skin texture. With laser skin resurfacing, patients experience significant skin renewal with fewer side effects and shorter recovery times compared to invasive procedures.

However, optimal results often require multiple sessions, especially for more challenging skin concerns, and each session typically takes between 30 minutes and 2 hours, depending on the treatment area.

Brief History And Evolution Of Laser Treatments In Skincare

Laser treatments in skincare began in the 1960s with the advent of the CO_2 laser, primarily used in medical treatments. This early laser type was powerful but imprecise for aesthetic use.

In the 1990s, dermatologists refined laser technology, allowing for controlled removal of skin layers to treat wrinkles, scars, and pigmentation, which laid the foundation for laser skin resurfacing.

As technology evolved, fractional lasers emerged, delivering targeted results with less recovery time by treating small skin areas at once.

The evolution from ablative to non-ablative lasers transformed skincare. Ablative lasers, such as CO_2 and Erbium lasers, remove skin layers and treat deeper wrinkles and scars. Non-ablative lasers, like Nd

and IPL, work beneath the skin's surface, promoting collagen without damaging the top layer. Fractional lasers, introduced in the early 2000s, allowed for skin healing between treated and untreated zones, making treatments more comfortable with reduced downtime.

Today, laser technology in skincare is advanced, offering tailored treatments to address specific skin concerns across a variety of skin types.

The evolution of lasers, including the development of pulsed dye and picosecond lasers, has expanded options to treat pigmentation, scars, and aging without lengthy recovery periods. Patients can now choose treatments based on recovery time, skin type, and targeted results, highlighting how far laser technology has come in making cosmetic treatments safer and more effective.

Types Of Skin Concerns Treated By Laser Resurfacing

Laser skin resurfacing can treat a wide range of skin issues, including fine lines, wrinkles, acne scars, sun damage, and uneven skin tone. It is effective in addressing hyperpigmentation issues, such as melasma and age spots, as well as tightening sagging skin.

By targeting the layers of skin where damage is present, laser resurfacing stimulates collagen production and accelerates cell turnover, making it an excellent option for skin rejuvenation and repair.

There are different types of lasers designed for specific skin concerns. For instance, fractional CO_2 lasers are commonly used for deeper wrinkles and significant skin damage, while Erbium lasers are effective for moderate resurfacing and fewer side effects.

For pigmentation issues, pulsed dye or Q-switched lasers are typically used, as they target melanin without affecting surrounding skin tissue. Dermatologists select the laser type based on the specific skin issue, depth, and desired recovery time.

Laser skin resurfacing is suitable for most common skin conditions; however, it is especially beneficial for individuals with visible signs of aging or scarring.

People with lighter skin tones often see the best results, as certain lasers can lead to pigmentation changes in darker skin.

Patients should discuss their skin concerns and history with a dermatologist to identify the best approach, ensuring optimal and safe results from their laser resurfacing treatment.

Benefits Of Laser Resurfacing For Different Skin Types

Laser skin resurfacing offers tailored benefits depending on skin type, including wrinkle reduction, skin tightening, and scar minimization.

For individuals with fair to medium skin tones, laser treatments can provide uniform results without high risks of pigmentation issues. Non-ablative lasers, which don't affect the surface layer, are beneficial for darker skin tones, minimizing the risk of hyperpigmentation and allowing even tone correction.

The treatment also caters to various levels of skin sensitivity and thickness. For example, people with sensitive skin might prefer fractional or non-ablative lasers, which are gentler on the surface and reduce the chance of irritation. Those with thicker or scarred skin often benefit from CO_2 or Erbium lasers, as they target deeper layers and provide more intensive treatment, ideal for deeper wrinkles or acne scars.

Each laser type can be customized based on the patient's needs, allowing for unique benefits like smoother texture and even pigmentation. Treatments can address specific needs in different areas, such as improving eye or lip areas with fine lasers.

A dermatologist will help select the best laser type and intensity for a patient's skin type, ensuring effective results that cater to individual needs and minimize recovery time.

Who Can Benefit Most From Laser Skin Resurfacing

Laser skin resurfacing is ideal for individuals seeking to improve the texture, tone, and appearance of their skin without invasive surgery. It benefits those with signs of aging, including wrinkles and fine lines, as well as people with acne scars, sun damage, or pigmentation irregularities. Patients with fair to medium skin tones tend to achieve the most consistent results due to a reduced risk of pigmentation issues associated with certain laser types.

The treatment is also beneficial for people who want a non-surgical method to achieve skin tightening and a youthful appearance. Those looking to address acne scarring, particularly atrophic scars, often find that laser resurfacing offers noticeable improvement. Patients with mature skin can benefit from the collagen-boosting effects of laser treatment, as it helps restore skin elasticity and minimizes age-related sagging.

However, laser resurfacing is not suited for everyone. Patients with active acne or certain medical conditions, like autoimmune disorders, may need to explore alternative treatments. A consultation with a dermatologist will help determine if laser resurfacing is appropriate, based on individual skin needs, medical history, and aesthetic goals.

CHAPTER TWO

Types Of Laser Resurfacing Techniques

Laser skin resurfacing techniques can vary widely depending on the depth of skin treatment, the type of laser used, and the desired results. The primary types include ablative lasers, which remove the top layer of skin for more dramatic effects, and non-ablative lasers, which work beneath the surface to stimulate collagen production without removing skin layers.

Ablative techniques are typically used for more severe skin issues, like deep wrinkles or scars, while non-ablative options are better suited for mild to moderate concerns.

CO_2 and erbium lasers are the most commonly used ablative lasers. CO_2 lasers are effective for deeper wrinkles and skin irregularities due to their intensity, while erbium lasers are more gentle, and often used for fine lines and mild scars. Fractional lasers, a more advanced option, can be either ablative or non-ablative. These lasers divide the light into thousands of tiny beams, treating small "fractions" of the skin at a time. This technique minimizes downtime while still providing noticeable results.

Finally, there's the pulsed-dye laser (PDL) and intense pulsed light (IPL), which technically aren't lasers but are used in resurfacing for pigmentation issues and redness.

While PDL is used for blood vessel-related concerns, IPL addresses pigment and is especially effective on lighter skin tones. Each technique serves specific purposes, and understanding these options helps tailor treatments for individual skin concerns.

CO_2 Lasers: How They Work And Their Benefits

CO_2 lasers are known for their intensity, making them a popular choice for treating deep wrinkles, severe sun damage, and other prominent skin irregularities. These lasers work by emitting short pulses of high-energy light that target water in skin cells, effectively vaporizing the outer skin layer. This controlled removal of the top skin layer stimulates the body's natural healing process, promoting collagen production, and giving way to smoother, firmer skin as it heals.

The CO_2 laser is a more aggressive option, ideal for people with significant skin issues who desire more transformative results. Patients often need local anesthesia or a numbing cream due to the intensity, and recovery can take one to two weeks. During this time, it's important to follow specific aftercare instructions, including applying prescribed ointments and avoiding sun exposure, to protect the healing skin and optimize results.

CO_2 laser treatment results can be long-lasting, with improvements noticeable even a few months post-treatment as collagen continues to rebuild.

However, the procedure does come with a risk of side effects like redness, swelling, and potential scarring, so it's essential to consult a qualified dermatologist to discuss suitability and manage expectations.

Erbium Lasers: Applications And Specific Skin Concerns

Erbium lasers provide a gentler alternative to CO_2 lasers, making them an excellent choice for treating fine lines, mild wrinkles, and shallow scars, particularly in sensitive areas like the face, neck, and chest. This laser targets water in the skin similarly to CO_2 lasers, but at a shallower depth, allowing for a more controlled, precise treatment that generally requires less downtime. This makes erbium laser resurfacing appealing for individuals looking for effective yet less intense skin renewal.

The healing period for erbium laser treatments is typically shorter, usually around a few days to a week, as it impacts fewer skin layers. Redness and peeling can still occur but are less pronounced than with more aggressive laser types. This gentler approach is also less likely to cause pigmentation changes, making it suitable for lighter and darker skin tones alike. For patients seeking minor enhancements with lower risk, erbium lasers are a practical option.

Erbium lasers are particularly effective for younger patients who may not yet have deep wrinkles or extensive skin damage but want to maintain a youthful appearance.

Post-treatment, it's recommended to keep the skin moisturized and shielded from sun exposure, which can affect the healing process. The results can last for several months to years, especially when combined with a consistent skincare routine.

Fractional Lasers: Advantages And Uses

Fractional lasers provide a versatile option for resurfacing, targeting both surface and deeper skin layers without treating the entire area. They break up the laser energy into thousands of microscopic treatment zones, leaving portions of the skin untreated. This technique, known as fractional photothermolysis, speeds up healing and minimizes recovery time, making it ideal for those with busy lifestyles who want noticeable results without significant downtime.

Fractional lasers are commonly used to improve skin texture, reduce fine lines, and treat mild scars. Depending on the intensity—either ablative or non-ablative—fractional lasers can address various skin concerns, from light resurfacing to deep remodeling.

Ablative fractional lasers are more effective for severe skin issues, but they come with more downtime, whereas non-ablative versions require less recovery, ideal for subtle enhancements.

Patients can often resume daily activities within a few days of fractional laser treatment, although some redness and peeling may occur. Since fractional lasers are customizable, they're often a good fit for people with multiple skin concerns. However, it's crucial to follow aftercare instructions to protect the treated areas, including regular moisturizing and sunscreen use, as the skin will be more sensitive post-treatment.

Non-Ablative Vs. Ablative Laser Treatments Explained

Ablative and non-ablative lasers represent the two main categories of laser treatments, each offering distinct benefits based on treatment needs and desired outcomes.

Ablative lasers remove the top layer of skin, making them more effective for treating deep wrinkles, acne scars, and sun damage.

They involve more downtime but can achieve dramatic improvements with fewer sessions, often requiring only one or two treatments for noticeable results.

Non-ablative lasers, on the other hand, work below the skin surface without removing layers. This stimulates collagen growth and repairs tissue gradually, making it an excellent choice for those with milder concerns, like fine lines or pigmentation issues, who prefer a gentler approach. Non-ablative treatments require multiple sessions but have minimal recovery time, allowing patients to return to regular activities quickly.

When choosing between these options, consider factors like age, skin type, lifestyle, and specific skin concerns.

While ablative treatments provide more noticeable results in one session, non-ablative treatments build up improvements over time. Consulting with a professional is crucial to weigh the pros and cons based on individual skin characteristics and treatment goals.

How To Choose The Right Laser For Individual Skin Needs

Selecting the right laser for skin resurfacing involves assessing specific skin concerns, skin type, and desired results. Individuals with deep wrinkles or significant skin damage often benefit more from ablative treatments, like CO_2 lasers, as they offer more powerful results. For milder issues, such as light pigmentation or early signs of aging, non-ablative options may be preferable as they involve less downtime and are gentler on the skin.

Patients with sensitive or darker skin types need to be cautious, as some lasers can increase pigmentation risks. Erbium lasers and non-ablative fractional lasers are often safer options in these cases, providing effective results without affecting skin tone.

Consulting with a licensed dermatologist or skincare professional can help evaluate which laser treatment aligns best with personal skin goals and reduce the risk of side effects.

Lifestyle factors, like the time available for recovery, should also influence the choice. For those unable to accommodate extended downtime, fractional or non-ablative lasers may be better suited. Ultimately, a thorough consultation that considers skin condition, type, and individual expectations will guide the selection process, ensuring the best possible results with minimized risks.

CHAPTER THREE

Preparing For Laser Resurfacing Treatment

Before undergoing laser skin resurfacing, preparing properly is crucial to achieve the best results and minimize risks. A good initial step is a comprehensive consultation with a qualified dermatologist or laser specialist. In this meeting, the provider will discuss your skin concerns, treatment goals, and any prior skin conditions or treatments. This is also the time to ask questions regarding the types of lasers available, the estimated downtime, and the number of sessions needed to achieve your desired results. The consultation helps to set clear expectations and ensure that laser resurfacing aligns with your skin's needs and your lifestyle.

Following this, a skin assessment and patch test are essential steps. The specialist will assess your skin type, tone, and texture to determine the appropriate laser type and intensity. During a patch test, a small area of skin is treated to monitor how your skin reacts to the laser, reducing the risk of adverse effects. This preliminary test allows the dermatologist to customize the treatment settings, ensuring it's safe and effective for you while reducing potential irritation or complications.

Pre-treatment skincare is key in laser resurfacing preparation. You may be advised to stop using certain products, like retinoids, alpha hydroxy acids, or exfoliants, as these can increase skin sensitivity.

It's also recommended to avoid sun exposure, as tanned skin may be more prone to burns or hyperpigmentation post-treatment. Your dermatologist might suggest specific cleansers, moisturizers, and sunscreens to prepare and strengthen your skin.

Avoiding these products and adopting protective routines will contribute to an optimal treatment outcome.

Initial Consultation: What To Expect And Questions To Ask

The initial consultation is an opportunity to gather all the information you need to make an informed decision about laser resurfacing.

During this appointment, your dermatologist will evaluate your skin concerns and go over your medical history to check for any contraindications. They may explain the different types of lasers used for resurfacing, such as ablative or non-ablative lasers, each suited to different skin needs and recovery times. This consultation allows you to understand what the procedure entails and how it will address your specific skin goals.

Asking the right questions during the consultation can help you gain a better understanding of the procedure.

Consider asking about the expected results, potential side effects, the estimated healing time, and the long-term maintenance required after the treatment.

It's also useful to ask about the recommended laser type for your skin type, the level of pain involved, and how to manage any discomfort during and after the procedure. These questions will help clarify any concerns you might have and set realistic expectations for the results.

Additionally, discussing the financial aspects of laser resurfacing, such as the cost per session and any package discounts, can be helpful. Some treatments may require multiple sessions for optimal results, so it's important to understand the full scope of investment. Understanding the costs involved, including follow-up appointments, allows you to make an informed decision and prepare for the journey ahead.

Skin Assessments And Patch Testing

A thorough skin assessment helps ensure a safe and effective laser treatment tailored to your unique skin profile. During this assessment, your dermatologist will examine your skin type, tone, sensitivity, and any areas of concern such as pigmentation, scars, or fine lines. This evaluation guides the choice of laser and helps to customize the treatment plan according to your specific needs, providing more accurate, effective results.

Patch testing is a crucial step to check how your skin will react to the laser before committing to the full treatment. A small, discreet area of your skin is treated, and you may need to wait for 24-48 hours to observe any reactions such as redness, swelling, or pigmentation changes. Patch tests help reduce the risk of adverse reactions during the actual procedure by allowing the dermatologist to adjust the laser settings based on your skin's response, ensuring a safe and effective treatment.

Your skin type and condition will also determine the pre-treatment recommendations that the dermatologist may suggest. For instance, those with more sensitive skin may need extra hydration and barrier-strengthening products, while others may need a regimen focused on calming inflammation. This assessment sets the foundation for a treatment plan designed to maximize benefits while minimizing discomfort or risks during the laser resurfacing procedure.

Pre-Treatment Skincare Routines And Products To Avoid

Preparing your skin for laser resurfacing involves following a skincare routine that strengthens and protects it ahead of treatment. Dermatologists often recommend using gentle cleansers and rich moisturizers to support skin hydration, ensuring your skin barrier is healthy and resilient.

Sun protection is vital, and applying a broad-spectrum sunscreen daily reduces the risk of hyperpigmentation after the procedure, as sun exposure can make skin more vulnerable to pigmentation changes.

Several skincare products should be avoided in the weeks leading up to your treatment. Retinoids, exfoliating acids (such as AHAs and BHAs), and certain active ingredients can increase skin sensitivity and should be paused. Additionally, avoid products with alcohol or fragrances that could lead to irritation. Switching to a gentle, hydrating routine will ensure your skin is calm and ready for treatment, reducing the risk of inflammation or discomfort.

Lastly, you might be instructed to stop using certain medications that can increase photosensitivity, such as specific antibiotics or anti-inflammatory drugs.

Your dermatologist will advise on any other restrictions, such as avoiding facial waxing or chemical peels.

By adhering to these skincare adjustments, you are actively setting the stage for a smoother, more effective laser resurfacing experience.

Lifestyle And Diet Adjustments Before The Procedure

Certain lifestyle and diet adjustments can help prepare your body and skin for laser resurfacing, ensuring better results and a faster recovery.

Reducing alcohol and caffeine intake in the days leading up to the procedure can decrease skin dryness and reduce the risk of increased sensitivity during treatment. Staying hydrated by drinking plenty of water supports skin health, helping it remain resilient and aiding in the healing process post-treatment.

A balanced diet rich in antioxidants, vitamins, and minerals can further support skin healing and collagen production. Foods high in vitamin C, such as citrus fruits, and those rich in omega-3 fatty acids, like salmon or flaxseeds, promote skin elasticity and resilience.

Avoiding processed foods and refined sugars can also minimize inflammation, setting the stage for a smoother recovery and more radiant skin post-treatment.

Your dermatologist may also suggest avoiding intense physical activities right before treatment, as sweating or heavy exercise can increase blood flow to the skin and heighten sensitivity during the procedure. Implementing these lifestyle modifications ahead of time ensures that your body and skin are in the best possible state for laser resurfacing, helping to achieve optimal, lasting results.

Understanding Treatment Risks And Potential Side Effects

Understanding the risks and potential side effects associated with laser resurfacing allows you to be fully prepared for the recovery process and any short-term changes in your skin's appearance. Common side effects may include redness, swelling, and mild discomfort, similar to a sunburn sensation, which usually subsides within a few days to weeks.

However, knowing what to expect can help ease any anxiety about these reactions and allow you to plan for recovery.

More serious but less common risks can include hyperpigmentation, scarring, or infection if post-care instructions aren't carefully followed. These risks are minimized by choosing an experienced dermatologist, undergoing a proper patch test, and adhering to pre- and post-treatment care.

Your dermatologist will guide you on proper post-care, which typically involves keeping the skin clean, hydrated, and protected from sunlight to avoid complications.

In some cases, the skin may take on a rougher texture or peel as it heals and rejuvenates.

By staying informed of these possibilities and following your dermatologist's guidance, you can ensure that any side effects are managed smoothly, ultimately leading to the glowing, rejuvenated results laser resurfacing is known for.

CHAPTER FOUR

Step-By-Step Laser Resurfacing Procedure

Laser skin resurfacing begins with a thorough cleaning of the skin to remove any oils, dirt, and makeup. Next, a topical numbing cream or local anesthetic is applied to reduce discomfort during the procedure, especially for high-energy lasers that reach deeper skin layers.

After the numbing agent has taken effect, the laser device is set to a specific wavelength based on the patient's skin type and treatment goals, such as wrinkle reduction or scar improvement. The practitioner then carefully directs the laser over the treatment area, often following a grid-like pattern to ensure even coverage and prevent overlap.

During the procedure, the laser emits short, concentrated light beams to target and remove damaged skin cells layer by layer.

Some lasers also create controlled "micro-injuries" to stimulate collagen production and skin renewal. The provider usually makes multiple passes over the skin, adjusting the laser settings as needed to treat different layers and areas. A cooling device or gel is sometimes used in tandem with the laser to keep the skin's surface from overheating and reduce discomfort, especially for non-ablative lasers, which focus on deeper skin layers without removing the top layer.

After the treatment, a soothing ointment or serum is applied to help with healing and reduce redness. A dressing or a cooling pad may be placed over the skin briefly to minimize initial swelling and soreness. Patients receive detailed aftercare instructions, including advice on gentle cleansing, moisturizing, and avoiding sun exposure. Following these steps ensures that the treated skin can heal properly and results in smoother, rejuvenated skin.

What Happens During A Typical Laser Resurfacing Session

Before the laser treatment begins, patients typically have a pre-procedure consultation where the provider explains the process and answers questions.

On the day of the session, the patient is settled comfortably in a treatment chair, and protective eyewear is provided to shield the eyes from the laser light. The practitioner preps the skin by cleaning and may apply a topical anesthetic or cooling gel, depending on the laser type and patient's comfort needs.

As the session starts, the provider uses a handheld laser device, which is carefully moved across the skin's surface. Each pulse of the laser targets specific skin cells or tissue, usually creating a slight tingling or warm sensation. The duration of each pass varies based on the type of laser and area treated. Some treatments require multiple passes over the same area to achieve the desired depth of skin renewal. Between passes, the provider may use a cool-air device to soothe the skin.

After the final pass, a calming serum or ointment is applied to soothe any immediate irritation. The skin may feel sensitive, warm, or tingly for a few hours post-session, but these effects generally subside. The provider gives aftercare guidance, such as applying a gentle moisturizer, avoiding harsh products, and protecting the skin from sun exposure to promote optimal healing and reduce the risk of complications.

Pain Management Options And What To Expect During Treatment

Laser skin resurfacing can involve some discomfort, but various pain management techniques help make the experience more tolerable. For lighter resurfacing treatments, a topical numbing cream is often sufficient, applied about 30–45 minutes before the procedure to reduce surface-level pain. For more intensive treatments, like CO_2 or erbium lasers, the provider might suggest a local anesthetic or nerve block, especially if large areas are being treated.

Some clinics also offer nitrous oxide (laughing gas) or oral sedatives to help patients feel relaxed and manage anxiety or discomfort. These options help make the procedure smoother, especially for patients nervous about potential pain. Advanced lasers may also have integrated cooling technology to reduce the skin's heat sensation during treatment.

Discussing these options with a provider before the session ensures that patients have the best comfort strategy for their needs.

Patients can expect a range of sensations during treatment, from mild tingling to intense warmth or a rubber-band snap feeling on the skin. Post-procedure, the skin may feel sensitive and tender, similar to a mild sunburn. Pain usually lessens within a day, and over-the-counter pain relievers and cold compresses are often recommended to ease any lingering discomfort.

The specific pain management plan should align with the type of laser used and the individual's comfort preferences.

Key Steps And Timeline Of The Procedure

Laser resurfacing typically follows a specific timeline, beginning with a pre-procedure consultation where the skin type, condition, and treatment goals are evaluated. The treatment usually starts with skin cleansing and the application of a topical anesthetic, which takes about 30–45 minutes to take effect. After numbing, the laser treatment itself can take 20–90 minutes, depending on the size of the treatment area and the depth required.

The laser session itself involves moving the device over the skin in a structured, overlapping pattern to ensure comprehensive coverage. This phase is relatively quick for small areas, like around the eyes or mouth, but can extend to an hour or more for larger sections, such as the entire face. As each laser pass is completed, the provider may apply cooling measures to the treated skin, particularly for intense, deep-resurfacing treatments.

Following the procedure, patients usually experience immediate redness and some swelling, which can last for several hours or up to a few days, depending on the laser type. Initial recovery can take 1–2 weeks, with visible improvements in skin tone and texture typically appearing within a month as the skin regenerates.

Patients should follow a post-procedure plan, including moisturizing and sun protection, to maximize results and protect the new skin.

Differences In Procedure Duration For Various Laser Types

Laser resurfacing duration varies widely based on the laser type, treatment area, and depth of skin penetration. Non-ablative lasers like fractional lasers are generally quicker, taking about 15–30 minutes per session, as they only treat the deeper layers without removing the top skin layer. This type of laser is often ideal for minor touch-ups, wrinkle softening, and treating minor scars and discolorations, making it a faster option with shorter recovery.

Ablative lasers, like CO_2 and erbium lasers, involve removing the top layers of skin, requiring more passes over the skin surface. Ablative treatments can take up to 1–2 hours for a full-face session due to the deeper, more intensive work involved. Fractional ablative lasers, which target specific zones while leaving surrounding skin intact, take less time than full ablative lasers but still require more time than non-ablative options.

For larger areas or combination treatments, the session duration can be extended, and the practitioner may use a mix of laser types for customized results. Each type of laser and treatment goal dictates not only the time spent but also the necessary recovery period. It's important to factor in both the time in-office and the healing time afterward when planning for laser resurfacing.

Tips For Staying Calm And Comfortable Throughout

To stay calm during laser skin resurfacing, consider deep breathing exercises or gentle meditation before the procedure. Bringing a supportive friend or family member can help reduce pre-treatment jitters. Talking with the provider about pain management and asking questions before the session also helps patients feel more informed and in control, reducing anxiety.

Distraction techniques, like listening to music or using calming scents, can also make the experience smoother. Many clinics provide earbuds or relaxing playlists to help patients feel more at ease during treatment. Taking slow, deep breaths during the session, especially if there is any discomfort, can help keep the body relaxed. Patients should communicate any concerns to their provider, as adjustments can often be made to enhance comfort. Post-treatment, gentle skincare, and cold compresses provide physical comfort while staying hydrated and resting helps the skin heal.

Following aftercare instructions precisely also builds confidence that recovery will proceed as planned. Knowing what to expect both during and after the session minimizes worry, allowing patients to feel prepared and positive about the outcome.

CHAPTER FIVE

Aftercare Essentials And Recovery Tips

Laser skin resurfacing requires careful aftercare to maximize results and ensure safe recovery. Immediately after treatment, your skin will be more sensitive, so prioritize gentle, nourishing skincare. Cleanse the treated area with lukewarm water and a mild, fragrance-free cleanser to avoid irritation. Avoid touching or scratching, as this can slow healing or lead to infection. Additionally, applying a gentle moisturizer or healing ointment helps lock in moisture, aiding skin regeneration and minimizing dryness. Hydration is also crucial, so drink plenty of water to help keep your skin resilient and supple.

Sun protection is paramount post-laser treatment as your skin will be more prone to sunburn and hyperpigmentation.

Avoid direct sun exposure as much as possible and always use a high SPF sunscreen (SPF 30 or higher) when stepping outdoors, even on cloudy days. Physical barriers, like hats and scarves, are also recommended to provide additional protection. Reapply sunscreen every two hours if you'll be outside for extended periods, as proper sun protection can significantly improve your laser treatment outcomes.

Consider using soothing products specifically formulated for sensitive skin to prevent further irritation during recovery. A gentle, non-abrasive moisturizer and a minimalistic approach to skincare reduce the risk of reactions. Avoid using active ingredients like retinoids, acids, or alcohol-based products for a few weeks until the skin is fully healed. Consulting with your skincare provider about the best post-care products and routines can also provide added guidance.

Immediate Post-Treatment Care: Do's And Don'ts

Immediately following laser skin resurfacing, adhere to a few essential "do's" to support healing. First, use a gentle, non-friction cleansing technique with lukewarm water and a fragrance-free cleanser. Pat dry with a soft towel instead of rubbing to avoid aggravating the treated skin. Applying a soothing, fragrance-free moisturizer or an ointment like petroleum jelly will help prevent dryness and promote healing by keeping the skin barrier intact.

There are also important "don'ts" to be aware of during this sensitive period. Avoid picking, scratching, or peeling the skin to prevent scarring and infection, as tempting as it might be when your skin feels dry or flaky. Avoid makeup for at least a few days post-treatment, as products could clog pores or irritate raw skin. Avoid hot showers, saunas, or any intense heat exposure as it can worsen redness and prolong recovery.

To further reduce the risk of complications, keep your skincare routine minimal. Don't use exfoliants, acids, or active treatments like retinol for a few weeks, as these can be too harsh. Avoid sun exposure, opting for a high-SPF sunscreen and physical barriers if you must go outside. Consulting with your dermatologist about approved products is also a great step toward safe recovery.

Recommended Skincare Products And Routines

A gentle, hydrating cleanser is ideal post-treatment. Look for one that is fragrance-free and formulated for sensitive skin to avoid irritation. Gentle foaming or cream-based cleansers without harsh surfactants help maintain the skin's natural barrier without stripping moisture.

Use lukewarm water and a soft washcloth to gently pat dry after cleansing, preventing friction or pressure on the treated areas.

Moisturizers are essential to lock in hydration and create a protective barrier on the skin. Opt for a thick, hypoallergenic cream or an ointment like petroleum jelly that can protect against dryness and help the skin repair itself. For daytime use, choose a moisturizer that contains broad-spectrum SPF 30 or higher to shield skin from sun exposure. If your skincare provider recommends it, consider adding a calming serum with soothing ingredients, like aloe vera or green tea, to reduce redness and inflammation.

During recovery, keep the routine simple and avoid active ingredients that could disrupt healing. Avoid products with alcohol, retinoids, or acids, as these can worsen irritation. If you have specific concerns, like post-treatment pigmentation or redness, consult your dermatologist about specialized creams that can be introduced once the initial healing is complete. Proper hydration, both internally and externally, also aids in faster recovery and lasting results.

Managing Pain, Swelling, And Redness Effectively

After laser resurfacing, you may experience some discomfort, including mild pain, swelling, and redness. Over-the-counter pain relievers, such as ibuprofen, can help manage any discomfort if recommended by your dermatologist. Cool compresses or ice packs can be used for a few minutes at a time to alleviate swelling, but always wrap them in a soft cloth to prevent direct contact with your skin.

Applying a calming ointment or a fragrance-free healing cream can reduce redness and swelling by soothing the treated area. Ingredients like aloe vera, panthenol, and chamomile have anti-inflammatory properties that help calm irritated skin. Remember to keep the area well-hydrated, as dryness can exacerbate redness and discomfort. Drink plenty of water throughout the day, as hydrated skin heals more efficiently and retains elasticity.

Redness and swelling may last for a few days to a couple of weeks, depending on the depth of your treatment.

If symptoms persist or worsen, contact your dermatologist, as this may indicate an allergic reaction or infection. Following your skin care provider's aftercare instructions and avoiding heavy products or makeup until full recovery can greatly reduce these side effects.

Expected Recovery Timeline And Stages Of Skin Healing

The initial recovery period after laser skin resurfacing is typically about one to two weeks, but this varies depending on treatment depth and individual skin type. In the first few days, you may experience redness, swelling, and tenderness, similar to a sunburn. During this stage, your skin will be most sensitive, so follow all aftercare instructions and avoid any harsh products or excessive sun exposure.

As you approach the one-week mark, you may notice flaking or peeling, which indicates that old, damaged skin is shedding to reveal newer skin beneath. Avoid picking or peeling off the flakes to allow your skin to heal naturally. A gentle moisturizer can keep the area hydrated and soothe irritation. Swelling and redness should gradually subside, though a light pink tint may remain on the skin for several weeks as healing continues.

Complete healing can take several weeks, with full results visible around the two-to-three-month mark for deeper treatments. During this period, continue to use sun protection and a gentle skincare routine. Over time, your skin should appear smoother, with improved texture and tone.

Consulting with your dermatologist about touch-up treatments or specialized serums can further enhance and maintain results.

Avoiding Sun Exposure And Protective Measures

Avoiding sun exposure is critical after laser skin resurfacing, as the skin becomes highly vulnerable to UV damage, which can lead to hyperpigmentation and other complications. For the first two weeks post-treatment, stay indoors as much as possible and avoid peak sunlight hours (10 a.m. to 4 p.m.) if you must be outside. If exposure is unavoidable, wear broad-brimmed hats and protective clothing for added safety. Sunscreen is essential, even when you're indoors, as UV rays can penetrate windows. Choose a high-SPF (30 or above), broad-spectrum sunscreen designed for sensitive or post-treatment skin. Physical sunscreens containing zinc oxide or titanium dioxide are especially effective and less likely to irritate. Apply generously and reapply every two hours if you're spending prolonged time outdoors.

To maintain and prolong results, prioritize sun protection as an integral part of your daily routine, even months after treatment. Applying sunscreen every morning and wearing protective accessories can help prevent pigmentation and preserve the smooth texture achieved through laser resurfacing. Taking these preventive measures will keep your skin healthy and your results vibrant for longer.

CHAPTER SIX

Long-Term Maintenance And Results

How Long Results Typically Last For Different Treatments

Laser skin resurfacing results depend on the type of laser used. Ablative lasers, like CO_2 and Erbium lasers, often provide dramatic improvements that can last several years since they target deeper layers of the skin. In contrast, non-ablative lasers such as Fraxel or IPL (Intense Pulsed Light) offer more subtle results that may last 6 to 12 months, requiring more frequent treatments to maintain the outcome.

Factors like age, skin type, and the initial skin concern can affect the duration of results. For example, treatments for fine lines or mild pigmentation may maintain results longer than treatments addressing deep wrinkles or severe sun damage.

As the skin continues to age naturally, the results will gradually fade, but the resurfacing slows the visible signs of aging.

Patients can expect the treated areas to improve further over the next 3 to 6 months post-treatment as collagen production increases. However, without proper follow-up care, environmental exposure (such as UV damage) can shorten the results.

Tips For Prolonging The Effects Of Laser Resurfacing

Daily sunscreen application with SPF 30+ is essential to protect treated skin from sun damage, which can prematurely age it and reverse laser results.

Using antioxidants, such as vitamin C serums, helps shield the skin from pollutants and free radicals. Moisturizers rich in hyaluronic acid will also keep the skin hydrated, promoting healing and preventing dryness or irritation.

Adopting a consistent skincare routine with retinoids or peptides can further stimulate collagen production, maintaining firmness and improving texture. Avoid smoking and limit alcohol consumption, as these habits can weaken skin elasticity and reduce the benefits of laser treatments. Additionally, following the post-procedure instructions from your provider ensures the healing process isn't interrupted.

It's also advisable to avoid harsh exfoliants or chemical peels for at least four weeks after treatment, as the skin remains sensitive. Staying hydrated, eating antioxidant-rich foods, and practicing good sleep hygiene will contribute to keeping the skin healthy and vibrant.

Maintenance Treatments: When And Why They're Needed

Even with a successful laser treatment, maintenance sessions may be required to prolong the results.

For non-ablative lasers, patients often undergo follow-up treatments every 6 to 12 months to maintain the effects. Ablative lasers usually require less frequent maintenance, with touch-ups recommended every 1 to 3 years depending on skin needs.

Maintenance sessions can help address new fine lines, minor pigmentation changes, or dullness that develop over time. They also serve to boost collagen production and prevent skin from losing elasticity. The need for additional treatments is determined by factors such as sun exposure, aging, and individual healing response.

A combination of procedures, such as microneedling or chemical peels, may complement the maintenance of laser resurfacing results. Consulting with your dermatologist ensures the ideal schedule is followed to preserve a youthful, refreshed appearance.

Importance Of Continued Skincare Routines

Maintaining an effective skincare routine post-laser treatment is critical for sustaining results. Cleansing the face gently and applying a soothing moisturizer helps restore the skin's barrier. Incorporating serums with ingredients like niacinamide and peptides can reduce inflammation and improve texture.

It's essential to protect the skin from harmful UV rays by using a broad-spectrum sunscreen daily. Sunscreen prevents hyperpigmentation and slows the reappearance of sun damage. Nightly use of retinoids or glycolic acids, under a dermatologist's guidance, can keep the skin smooth and promote long-term collagen production.

Skincare routines should adapt to the seasons; for example, richer moisturizers during winter and lighter products in summer.

Routine follow-ups with your dermatologist also allow adjustments to your regimen based on how the skin evolves.

Key Factors That Can Impact The Longevity Of Results

Several elements affect how long the benefits of laser resurfacing last. Sun exposure is a primary factor—unprotected UV exposure can lead to the reappearance of dark spots and wrinkles.

Skin type also plays a role; oily or acne-prone skin may require additional care to maintain results compared to dry skin types.

Lifestyle factors like smoking, excessive alcohol intake, and poor diet can accelerate aging and shorten the longevity of laser results. Conversely, healthy habits—such as a balanced diet, proper hydration, and regular sleep—contribute to skin longevity. Hormonal changes, especially during pregnancy or menopause, may also impact results.

Environmental exposure to pollutants and extreme weather can degrade the skin's quality over time.

Protective measures, including wearing hats, avoiding peak sun hours, and using barrier creams, can help maintain laser-treated skin's youthful appearance.

CHAPTER SEVEN

Common Concerns And Risks

Laser skin resurfacing can address many skin issues, but it also has certain risks and concerns that anyone considering the procedure should understand. One common concern is the possibility of skin discoloration, particularly for those with darker skin tones. Hyperpigmentation or hypopigmentation (darkening or lightening of the skin) can sometimes occur, so choosing a laser treatment suited to your skin type and following the proper aftercare is essential. Additionally, scarring is another risk, although rare with modern laser techniques. Consulting with an experienced dermatologist can minimize this risk by ensuring you're a suitable candidate for the procedure.

Infection prevention is a key consideration, as resurfacing temporarily removes the skin's outer layer, which can make it vulnerable.

To lower infection risks, providers recommend avoiding certain activities and products until the skin has healed. A clean, non-irritating moisturizer can keep the skin hydrated while it recovers, and some providers may prescribe topical antibiotics. It's also essential to monitor for signs of infection, such as unusual redness, warmth, or discharge, which, if noticed, should prompt a visit to the clinic.

Another concern is post-treatment redness, swelling, and skin sensitivity, which are common and typically short-lived. Redness can last a few weeks to months, depending on the intensity of the treatment. Applying soothing creams and following your doctor's recommendations can help manage these symptoms. For swelling, gentle cool compresses and sleeping with your head elevated may help. If results don't align with your expectations, speak with your provider, as there may be options for follow-up treatments or adjustments.

Understanding Hyperpigmentation And Scarring Risks

Hyperpigmentation, or darkening of the skin, is a frequent concern with laser resurfacing, especially for those with medium to darker skin tones. After the treatment, the skin may temporarily produce more melanin in response to the laser's heat. Choosing the right type of laser for your skin tone and a reputable provider can help minimize this risk. Doctors often recommend using a broad-spectrum sunscreen post-treatment to protect healing skin from UV exposure, which could otherwise trigger further pigmentation.

On the other hand, hypopigmentation, or lightening of the skin, can also occur. This is more common with more aggressive treatments, where deeper layers of skin are impacted.

Although rare, some people may experience permanent changes in pigmentation. To avoid this, providers may test a small skin area before proceeding and encourage treatments that gradually resurface the skin rather than intense, single treatments.

Scarring is less common but can occur if the skin is not adequately cared for during the healing process. Following post-care instructions carefully, such as avoiding picking at the skin or applying unapproved products, is critical. If scarring does occur, there are options to treat it, such as with follow-up laser treatments or certain creams that help reduce scar appearance.

Infection Prevention And Signs To Watch For

Preventing infection post-laser treatment is essential since laser resurfacing temporarily disrupts the skin barrier, making it vulnerable to bacteria.

Clean, gentle skincare practices, as well as avoiding makeup and other skin products on the treated area until it's healed, help reduce infection risks. Your doctor may also provide an antibacterial ointment to apply immediately after the procedure.

Recognizing the signs of infection early can prevent complications. Watch for symptoms like increased redness, tenderness, or unusual discharge from the treated area. Slight swelling or warmth is normal, but these should improve after the first few days. If the symptoms worsen, consult your provider promptly to ensure appropriate steps are taken.

Sticking to a gentle, fragrance-free moisturizer can help keep the skin hydrated without causing irritation or introducing bacteria. Some people choose to avoid public areas, saunas, and gyms immediately following treatment to minimize exposure to bacteria.

A mindful approach and communication with your dermatologist can greatly reduce the risk of post-treatment infections.

Addressing Redness, Swelling, And Sensitivity Post-Treatment

Redness, swelling, and sensitivity are common following laser skin resurfacing, and managing these side effects is essential for a smooth recovery. Redness can last from a few days to several weeks depending on the depth of the treatment, with deeper treatments causing more prolonged redness. To reduce irritation, many doctors recommend a hydrating, non-irritating cream that can soothe the skin without clogging pores.

Swelling, especially around the eyes or areas treated intensely, often peaks within the first 24–48 hours. To help alleviate swelling, apply a cold compress or ice wrapped in a clean cloth on the area. Sleeping with your head slightly elevated may also assist in reducing facial swelling overnight. Over-the-counter pain relievers, such as ibuprofen, may help with any discomfort, but consult your provider before taking any medication.

Sensitivity to sunlight and certain skincare products is normal post-treatment. It's essential to avoid direct sun exposure for several weeks following treatment and use a high-SPF sunscreen.

Harsh ingredients, such as retinoids, exfoliants, or alcohol-based products, should be avoided until the skin fully recovers. Gentle skincare, sun protection, and following aftercare guidelines will help soothe and protect your skin during this period.

What To Do If Results Aren't As Expected

Laser skin resurfacing is effective, but results may not always meet expectations immediately or entirely. If your results appear uneven or your skin doesn't heal as expected, consult your dermatologist for an assessment.

They may recommend additional treatments, such as light chemical peels or more laser sessions, to improve the overall result. In some cases, patience is key, as it can take weeks or even months for the full benefits to become evident.

If you're unhappy with certain aspects of the treatment, a follow-up consultation can help. Sometimes the skin requires more time to adjust, and your provider may suggest supportive skincare or specific products to enhance your results. Maintaining open communication with your provider is crucial to ensure that any necessary adjustments or additional care is provided.

Occasionally, certain skin types respond differently to laser resurfacing, leading to minor inconsistencies. Providers may use dermal fillers or additional laser sessions for correction. Remember that laser treatments often require a series of sessions to achieve optimal results, so it's essential to understand that achieving a fully transformed look may take time.

Myths Vs. Realities Of Laser Skin Resurfacing

One common myth is that laser resurfacing is painful and requires extensive downtime. In reality, most patients report mild discomfort that can be managed with topical numbing creams or, in more intensive cases, a local anesthetic. While deeper treatments can require a few days to a week for initial healing, many modern lasers minimize downtime and discomfort.

Another misconception is that laser resurfacing results are instant. Many assume that skin will look transformed immediately post-procedure, but visible improvement generally takes time as the skin heals and regenerates. Full results may take weeks or months to appear as collagen production increases and the skin renews. Patience is necessary, and realistic expectations can lead to more satisfaction with the gradual results.

Lastly, a common myth is that laser treatments are only suitable for those with lighter skin tones. With advances in laser technology, there are now safe and effective options for a range of skin types, including darker complexions. Consulting with an experienced provider familiar with different skin tones ensures that the appropriate laser and settings are chosen for optimal results without added risk.

CHAPTER EIGHT

Choosing The Right Clinic And Practitioner

Selecting a reputable clinic and practitioner for laser skin resurfacing is crucial to ensure a safe and effective treatment. Look for a certified dermatologist or plastic surgeon with specific expertise in laser treatments. Verify that the clinic is equipped with advanced, well-maintained laser devices, as outdated equipment can result in poor results or even complications.

Ensure that the staff is professional, knowledgeable, and willing to answer questions about their experience and training with laser skin resurfacing.

To verify credentials, check for board certification in dermatology or plastic surgery, as well as membership in recognized professional organizations like the American Board of Dermatology or the American Society for Laser Medicine and Surgery. Look for practitioners with a track record of performing laser treatments and ask to see before-and-after photos of previous clients to gauge the quality of their work. Online reviews and testimonials can also offer insights into the clinic's reputation and overall client satisfaction.

When selecting a clinic, prioritize facilities that offer personalized consultations and customized treatment plans. A thorough consultation is essential to discuss your skin type, goals, and any pre-existing conditions, ensuring that the procedure is tailored to your needs.

Avoid practitioners who make unrealistic promises, rush consultations, or push for unnecessary add-on services. Trustworthy clinics will take the time to assess your suitability for the procedure and educate you on the entire process, including potential risks and expected outcomes.

Qualities To Look For In A Laser Skin Resurfacing Specialist

A good laser skin resurfacing specialist should have extensive experience, a solid educational background, and a specific focus on laser treatments. Look for a professional who has not only completed medical training in dermatology or plastic surgery but has also pursued additional training in laser technology. This is important because laser treatments are highly specialized, and even experienced dermatologists need specific laser expertise to deliver safe and effective results.

The best practitioners are transparent, patient, and willing to discuss the entire procedure in detail, including potential side effects and aftercare requirements. They should ask about your medical history, skin type, and personal goals, and assess your skin's readiness for laser treatment. Ideally, the practitioner should conduct a small test patch on your skin to evaluate how it reacts to the laser before proceeding with full treatment.

Additionally, specialists who stay updated on the latest techniques and advancements in laser technology demonstrate a commitment to providing high-quality care. Continuous education and training mean they are likely aware of the safest, most effective methods available and can offer a broader range of treatment options. A dedicated laser specialist will also provide realistic expectations, aiming for gradual improvement rather than promising immediate or miraculous results.

How To Verify Credentials And Experience

Verifying the credentials and experience of a laser skin resurfacing specialist is essential to safeguard your skin and achieve the desired results. First, ensure that the practitioner is licensed by the appropriate medical board in your country and specializes in dermatology or plastic surgery. For example, in the U.S., you can use resources like the American Board of Medical Specialties to verify a provider's certification.

Checking for memberships in reputable professional organizations, such as the American Society for Laser Medicine and Surgery, is also beneficial. These memberships often require practitioners to meet high standards, which can assure you of their competency.

Ask about their experience with laser skin resurfacing specifically, including the types of lasers they use and how many treatments they have performed. A well-rounded specialist will have significant experience and a thorough understanding of the nuances involved in laser procedures.

If possible, request testimonials or view before-and-after photos of previous clients, which can provide insight into the specialist's skill level and treatment quality.

Additionally, don't hesitate to ask the practitioner to walk you through the procedure step-by-step during the consultation. An experienced and qualified specialist will have no problem addressing your concerns and ensuring you feel confident about moving forward.

Tips For Finding Trustworthy Clinics Near You

Finding a trustworthy laser skin resurfacing clinic near you begins with thorough research and recommendations. Start by searching for clinics with high ratings and positive reviews on reputable platforms, such as Google Reviews, Yelp, or RealSelf. Seeking personal recommendations from friends or family who have undergone laser treatments can also provide reliable insights. Pay attention to clinics with a long-standing reputation for quality and client satisfaction, as these are usually indicators of trustworthiness.

Once you have a shortlist, visit the clinics in person if possible to get a feel for their environment and staff professionalism. A reliable clinic will offer a clean, well-organized space and use state-of-the-art equipment. During your visit, inquire about the types of lasers they use and whether they offer different laser options to match various skin types. Clinics that focus solely on one or two laser machines might not have the versatility needed for optimal results.

It's essential to prioritize clinics that provide an initial consultation before any treatment. The consultation should be a thorough discussion of your skin type, goals, and medical history. Avoid any clinic that skips this step or doesn't provide a custom treatment plan. Clinics that pressure you to buy packages or promise guaranteed results should raise red flags, as these are often signs of profit-focused, rather than patient-centered, operations.

Importance Of A Thorough Consultation And Customized Plan

A thorough consultation and customized treatment plan are crucial steps in ensuring the safety and success of your laser skin resurfacing procedure.

During the consultation, the practitioner should assess your skin type, texture, and any underlying conditions to determine whether laser resurfacing is suitable. This step is essential because laser treatments are not ideal for everyone; factors like skin tone, medical history, and even lifestyle habits can impact the treatment's safety and effectiveness.

Customized treatment plans take into account individual skin concerns, such as acne scars, wrinkles, or pigmentation issues, tailoring the laser type and intensity to suit your needs. For instance, people with lighter skin tones may be good candidates for more aggressive lasers like CO_2, while those with darker skin tones may benefit from less intense lasers to avoid hyperpigmentation risks. A well-planned approach ensures that the treatment is as effective as possible with minimal risk of complications.

During the consultation, the practitioner should also discuss realistic expectations, potential risks, and aftercare instructions. The best specialists will explain what to expect during and after the procedure, including downtime and potential side effects.

This personalized, informative approach allows you to make an informed decision, reducing anxiety and increasing your confidence in the treatment process.

Red Flags To Avoid In A Practitioner Or Clinic

There are several red flags to watch out for when selecting a practitioner or clinic for laser skin resurfacing. One significant warning sign is a lack of board certification or specific experience in laser treatments.

Practitioners who are not certified in dermatology or plastic surgery, or who do not specialize in laser technology, may not have the knowledge needed to perform the procedure safely.

Another red flag is a clinic that does not offer an initial consultation or fails to inquire about your medical history and specific skin goals. Laser skin resurfacing requires a customized approach, and clinics that do not provide personalized treatment plans or pressure you into purchasing package deals may prioritize profits over client safety.

Avoid clinics that make unrealistic promises, such as guaranteed results or immediate transformations, as these claims are often misleading and may indicate a lack of professionalism.

Poor-quality or outdated equipment is also a cause for concern. Ensure that the clinic uses modern, FDA-approved lasers and that the machines are well-maintained.

Lastly, be wary of any clinic that does not provide comprehensive aftercare instructions, as proper post-treatment care is essential for achieving safe and effective results. The right clinic and practitioner will prioritize your well-being and provide all the necessary information for a successful experience.

CHAPTER NINE

Laser Skin Resurfacing For Different Skin Types

Laser skin resurfacing is customized to suit various skin types, ensuring safe and effective results. Skin types are primarily classified using the Fitzpatrick scale, which categorizes skin based on its reaction to sun exposure, ranging from very fair (Type I) to deeply pigmented (Type VI).

For lighter skin types (I-III), the risk of hyperpigmentation is lower, which allows for more aggressive treatments with higher energy levels. However, for darker skin types (IV-VI), lasers are used more cautiously to minimize the risk of pigmentation changes or scarring.

Knowing one's skin type is the first step in determining the appropriate laser treatment.

Different skin types also react to laser treatments uniquely. For example, lighter skin types may experience less downtime due to faster healing, while darker skin may require extended recovery. Dry or sensitive skin types can benefit from fractional lasers, which only treat a portion of the skin and allow faster recovery. Oily or acne-prone skin types may benefit from non-ablative lasers, which penetrate deeply to stimulate collagen without affecting the outer skin layer. Tailoring laser intensity and type-to-skin reaction helps minimize risks while maximizing results.

Personalizing laser resurfacing for sensitive or darker skin requires a gentler approach.

For those with sensitive skin, lasers that cause minimal thermal damage, like non-ablative lasers, are recommended. Darker skin tones may benefit from Nd

Lasers, which have a longer wavelength, reaching deeper layers while bypassing the melanin-rich outer layer. Patients with rosacea or acne scars may see results with fractional CO_2 or erbium lasers, which target deeper scars and reduce redness effectively, without over-exfoliating the skin surface.

Skin Type Considerations: Fitzpatrick Scale And Beyond

The Fitzpatrick Scale is essential for determining how skin types will respond to laser resurfacing. This scale ranges from Type I (very fair, burns easily) to Type VI (deeply pigmented, rarely burns), guiding treatment intensity and laser choice. For instance, Type I skin can withstand more intensive laser treatments as the risk of hyperpigmentation is low. In contrast, Types IV-VI, which include olive to dark skin tones, are more prone to pigmentation issues, thus needing gentler laser options to prevent post-inflammatory hyperpigmentation.

In addition to the Fitzpatrick Scale, individual characteristics like skin sensitivity, hydration level, and overall skin health are crucial in determining the best laser approach.

People with dry skin, for example, may require more hydration pre-treatment to avoid excessive irritation, while oily skin types might need lasers that also address acne control.

Skin conditions such as rosacea or eczema also require milder, non-ablative lasers to avoid flare-ups, helping to reduce inflammation without compromising skin integrity.

A personalized assessment considers factors beyond skin tone alone, such as genetic predispositions and lifestyle, which affect healing. Understanding these factors allows professionals to select a laser treatment plan that minimizes adverse effects. For instance, erbium or non-ablative lasers are effective for those prone to hyperpigmentation, while fractional lasers may suit those needing faster recovery. This approach ensures that the treatment aligns with both skin type and individual concerns, leading to safer and more satisfactory outcomes.

How Different Skin Types Respond To Laser Treatments

Each skin type responds differently to laser treatments, which is largely dictated by its pigment and texture. Lighter skin types tend to heal faster with fewer pigmentation concerns, making them suitable for intense treatments such as ablative CO_2 lasers, which target deep layers and renew the skin surface. However, darker skin types often react to heat by producing more pigment, posing a higher risk of hyperpigmentation and scarring if lasers are too aggressive. Consequently, for darker skin, gentler lasers like the Nd are often recommended, as they bypass the melanin-heavy outer layers.

Sensitive skin may be more prone to redness and irritation after laser resurfacing, so treatments are often spaced out and carefully monitored. For example, non-ablative lasers like IPL (Intense Pulsed Light) or erbium lasers work well for sensitive skin, targeting deeper skin layers without overheating the surface. People with dry skin may experience additional dryness post-treatment, making pre- and post-laser hydration crucial to prevent excessive peeling and irritation, often using hydrating serums or barrier repair creams to maintain balance.

For oily or acne-prone skin, lasers like fractional CO_2 or erbium are beneficial as they penetrate deeper layers, stimulating collagen without clogging pores.

These lasers can help reduce sebum production, contributing to fewer breakouts. The key to effective laser treatment is a thorough pre-treatment consultation to determine the optimal laser type and settings for each individual's unique skin profile. This personalized approach enhances results while minimizing adverse effects for various skin types.

Tailoring The Procedure For Sensitive Or Darker Skin Tones

For sensitive or darker skin tones, laser skin resurfacing must be carefully tailored to avoid side effects like hyperpigmentation or irritation. Darker skin tones are often best treated with longer-wavelength lasers, such as Nd, which penetrate deeper layers without disturbing melanin on the surface.

Sensitive skin, on the other hand, benefits from non-ablative lasers like erbium or IPL, which have lower heat levels and reduce the risk of post-treatment redness or inflammation.

To reduce discomfort for sensitive skin, a numbing cream is usually applied before laser resurfacing to minimize any discomfort. Treatments may also be spaced out to allow sufficient recovery time and prevent over-stressing the skin. Cooling devices during the procedure can further ease discomfort for sensitive or dark skin, helping to reduce inflammation and improve healing time.

Aftercare is especially important for these skin types, as both are prone to post-inflammatory hyperpigmentation.

A skincare routine that includes gentle, non-irritating moisturizers and SPF protection is essential for preventing dark spots and ensuring smooth, even healing. Following tailored protocols for darker and sensitive skin types allows clients to enjoy effective laser results without complications.

Choosing The Best Laser For Oily, Dry, Or Combination Skin

Selecting the appropriate laser for specific skin types, such as oily, dry, or combination skin, is crucial for achieving optimal results. Oily skin, for instance, may benefit from fractional lasers that can target the deeper skin layers, helping to balance oil production and reduce the appearance of pores. Fractional CO_2 or erbium lasers are often effective for oily skin as they stimulate collagen and improve skin texture without clogging pores. For those with acne-prone skin, combining laser resurfacing with blue light therapy can provide added benefits by reducing acne-causing bacteria.

For dry skin, non-ablative lasers like IPL or erbium work well as they are less intensive and do not strip moisture from the skin. Maintaining hydration is essential, so dry skin types should focus on using rich moisturizers both before and after the procedure. Some lasers also include a hydrating feature to replenish moisture levels during the process, preventing excessive dryness or peeling afterward.

Combination skin requires a more balanced approach, where different areas are treated according to their needs. Fractional lasers can provide a gentle overall treatment, targeting oilier areas with more energy while being cautious with drier patches. Customizing laser settings for each skin type ensures comfort and effective results, allowing individuals to achieve smoother, balanced skin post-treatment.

Managing Special Skin Concerns Like Acne Scars Or Rosacea

For those with specific skin concerns like acne scars or rosacea, laser skin resurfacing can offer significant improvements but requires a tailored approach. Acne scars often respond well to fractional CO_2 or erbium lasers, which target deeper skin layers to stimulate collagen production and smooth scarred tissue. These lasers help to reduce the appearance of pitted scars over multiple sessions, gradually creating a more even texture. For people with active acne, however, non-ablative lasers and light therapies that reduce bacteria may be preferable to avoid aggravating the skin.

Rosacea, on the other hand, demands a gentler touch as it involves sensitive blood vessels prone to redness. Lasers like IPL (Intense Pulsed Light) are often recommended for rosacea, as they can selectively target redness without heating the surrounding skin, reducing the risk of flare-ups. This type of laser minimizes rosacea's visible effects, leading to a more even skin tone and reducing facial redness over time.

For both conditions, post-treatment care includes avoiding harsh skincare products and using SPF daily to protect sensitive skin.

A series of treatments spaced over weeks or months provides gradual improvement, allowing skin time to adjust and heal between sessions. This incremental approach helps manage skin concerns effectively while minimizing irritation and downtime, especially for sensitive conditions like acne scars and rosacea.

CHAPTER TEN

Frequently Asked Questions (FAQs)

How Painful Is Laser Resurfacing?

Laser skin resurfacing can cause some discomfort, but the level of pain varies depending on the depth of the treatment and the individual's pain tolerance. For lighter, superficial treatments like non-ablative lasers, patients may only feel mild stinging or heat during the procedure. More aggressive treatments, such as ablative lasers that go deeper into the skin, can cause more intense discomfort. To ease this, topical numbing creams or local anesthesia are usually applied before the procedure.

During the treatment, many patients describe a sensation similar to a rubber band snapping against the skin, followed by a warm, sunburn-like feeling. Cooling devices are often used to soothe the skin as the laser works, helping to reduce discomfort. For deeper resurfacing treatments, some clinics may offer sedation or pain medications, so it's important to discuss pain management options with your provider beforehand.

Post-treatment discomfort is generally mild to moderate, with some redness, swelling, and tightness in the skin for a few days. Pain relievers and ice packs can help manage these symptoms during the recovery period. Aftercare, such as moisturizing and avoiding direct sunlight, also plays a key role in minimizing pain and aiding healing.

What Is The Ideal Age To Start Laser Treatments?

There is no specific age that is universally considered ideal for starting laser resurfacing treatments, as it depends more on the condition of the skin than on age. Generally, people in their 30s and 40s who are starting to notice early signs of aging, such as fine lines, wrinkles, or uneven skin tone, often seek laser treatments. However, some people in their 20s may opt for less aggressive, non-ablative lasers to address acne scars, and sun damage, or to maintain youthful skin.

Laser resurfacing can also be effective for older individuals looking to reduce deeper wrinkles, age spots, or sagging skin. The key is to customize the treatment based on individual skin needs and goals.

An evaluation by a dermatologist or cosmetic professional is crucial to determine the right time and type of laser treatment.

In essence, laser resurfacing isn't just age-dependent—it's more about addressing specific skin concerns. Whether you're looking to enhance your skin texture in your 20s or correct more advanced signs of aging in your 50s, laser treatments can be tailored accordingly.

Can Laser Resurfacing Be Combined With Other Treatments?

Yes, laser resurfacing can often be combined with other treatments for enhanced results, depending on your skin goals. For instance, many people choose to combine laser treatments with injectable fillers like Botox or dermal fillers to address both surface-level skin issues (such as texture and tone) and deeper concerns like volume loss or wrinkles. The combination allows for a more comprehensive rejuvenation of the face.

Another common pairing is with chemical peels or microneedling. These treatments work well together because laser resurfacing targets deeper layers of the skin, while a chemical peel or microneedling can boost collagen production and enhance surface exfoliation. However, it's important to space these treatments out properly and follow professional advice to avoid overloading your skin.

Your skincare provider will typically design a treatment plan that sequences these procedures safely and effectively. Combining treatments can maximize results and shorten the overall time needed to achieve your desired look, but it's essential to do so under the guidance of a qualified professional to minimize risks and ensure proper healing.

Will Insurance Cover Any Part Of Laser Resurfacing?

In most cases, insurance does not cover laser skin resurfacing, as it is typically considered a cosmetic procedure. Cosmetic treatments, including laser resurfacing, are seen as elective, and insurance providers usually won't cover them unless they are medically necessary. However, if the laser treatment is being used to treat a medical condition, such as severe acne scars or precancerous skin growths, there may be a possibility of partial coverage.

It's important to check with both your dermatologist and your insurance company to see if there's a chance that any part of the procedure could be covered. You may need to provide documentation that proves the treatment is medically necessary rather than purely cosmetic. Some patients have successfully received partial reimbursement for laser treatments related to specific health conditions, but this is generally the exception rather than the rule.

To avoid surprises, clarify all costs involved in the procedure before scheduling the treatment. Many cosmetic clinics offer payment plans or financing options to make the cost of laser resurfacing more manageable for those paying out of pocket.

How Soon Can Makeup Be Worn After The Procedure?

The timing for wearing makeup after laser resurfacing largely depends on the type of laser treatment you receive and how quickly your skin heals. For non-ablative laser treatments, which target the deeper layers of skin without removing the surface layer, you may be able to wear makeup within 24 to 48 hours. However, your skin may still be slightly red or sensitive, so it's important to use gentle, non-comedogenic makeup products that won't irritate your skin.

For ablative laser resurfacing, which removes layers of skin, the healing process is more extensive. Patients should typically wait at least 7 to 10 days before applying makeup. During this time, it's crucial to follow aftercare instructions, such as using prescribed ointments and avoiding sun exposure, to ensure the skin heals properly. Applying makeup too soon can hinder healing and may even increase the risk of infection.

Once your skin has fully healed and you've received the go-ahead from your dermatologist, opt for mineral-based makeup, as it is lighter and less likely to clog pores or cause irritation. Avoid heavy foundations and products with harsh chemicals, especially during the early stages of healing.

Conclusion

In conclusion, laser skin resurfacing techniques have transformed modern dermatology and aesthetic treatments, offering a range of options for improving skin texture, tone, and appearance. These techniques, including ablative, non-ablative, and fractional lasers, allow for tailored approaches based on individual skin concerns and conditions.

Ablative lasers, which include CO_2 and Erbium lasers, are highly effective for deep skin resurfacing, targeting wrinkles, scars, and other significant imperfections by removing the top layer of skin. Non-ablative lasers, such as intense pulsed light (IPL) and Nd

Lasers, stimulate collagen production beneath the skin without removing the outer layer, resulting in reduced downtime and a gentler recovery process. Fractional lasers combine the best of both methods by creating micro-wounds that promote collagen production while preserving surrounding skin areas, making it effective for both moderate and extensive rejuvenation.

Selecting the appropriate laser skin resurfacing technique depends on several factors, including the patient's skin type, the nature of skin concerns, desired results, and tolerance for recovery time. Consulting with a qualified dermatologist or aesthetic specialist is crucial to ensure the procedure aligns with the patient's goals and minimizes risks.

While the potential for improved skin appearance is high, patients should also be aware of the risks, such as pigmentation changes, scarring, and the need for sun protection post-procedure.

Laser skin resurfacing represents a powerful tool for achieving youthful, rejuvenated skin. As technology continues to advance, these techniques are becoming more effective, precise, and accessible. With the right guidance, patients can achieve significant improvements in skin quality and confidence, making laser skin resurfacing an invaluable option in skin care. Overall, laser skin resurfacing offers promising results for skin renewal and will likely continue to evolve as a cornerstone of skin rejuvenation therapies.

THE END

www.ingramcontent.com/pod-product-compliance
Lightning Source LLC
Chambersburg PA
CBHW052320220526
45472CB00001B/204